This book is dedicated to my dear grandmother who spent her life fighting for people like me, then took me in at eight months and raised me herself. She's the strongest person I know and I hope I'm making her proud every single day.

This book is also dedicated to black and brown women, rape and abuse survivors, fat women of color, disabled women of color, and people of color in the LGBT+ community.

Thank you for everything.

Table of Contents

Melt

Circles **(Trigger Warning: This Poem is About Abuse, Rape)**

Daffodils

Architect

Happy Place

Black Sappho

Dear Fat Girl

Rise

The Color Series
Purple

Blue

Green

Yellow

Orange

Red

Guest Poems
Struggle

Beckoning

routine.

Untitled

he?

Through The Mist

About The Artist

About The Author

MUD

The lotus flower asks permission from no one. Surrounded

by mud, buried beneath it, the lotus flower rises. It blooms

beautifully and unapologetically. Petals reaching for the sky, it is

once again victorious. The lotus has fought for this, lost once or

twice. It prevailed. The lotus stands for compassion, spiritual

awakening, intelligence, and rebirth. I hope, I too, can be

representative of these things to the people around me. I want to

be able to rise above my own murky waters and bloom

unapologetically.

All my life, I have struggled with an extensive and

life-altering medical history. The majority of my disabilities are

inherited. However, some of them were developed through

abusive relationships inside and outside of my family, my

environment, and were direct effects from an eating disorder I

suffered from. I had always thought my disabilities held me back until recently, when I decided that I deserved self compassion. I decided I could no longer put my health on the back burner for any reason. This has helped my health extensively. Although, I am still chronically ill, I now know to be kind to myself when there is no more I can do.

I have had to educate myself on many things from a young age on how my disabilities would affect me, my ethnicities, my cultures, and how to receive help for my family when my mother left my grandmother and I to care for my siblings. I was seven years old. I had to grow up quickly and learn that I did not have much time to be a child. There was not much time before I would be subject to racism, biphobia, sexism, ableism, and poverty. Education became a coping mechanism. It founded my hope and my hope for getting to a place where I would be able to help others like myself.

I was reborn after I escaped from an abusive relationship. I had decided to turn my pain into power. I learned a new language, became an activist, and moved out of state to get a head start on my degree. I was on a mission to become a new version of myself. A version that was powerful and someone I could be proud of when I looked at my reflection. I was always powerful, but, I had to make a habit of rebuilding myself; It became my only way of surviving.

I will rise above the mud and bloom unscathed. I will stretch my petals to the sun. I will win this war.

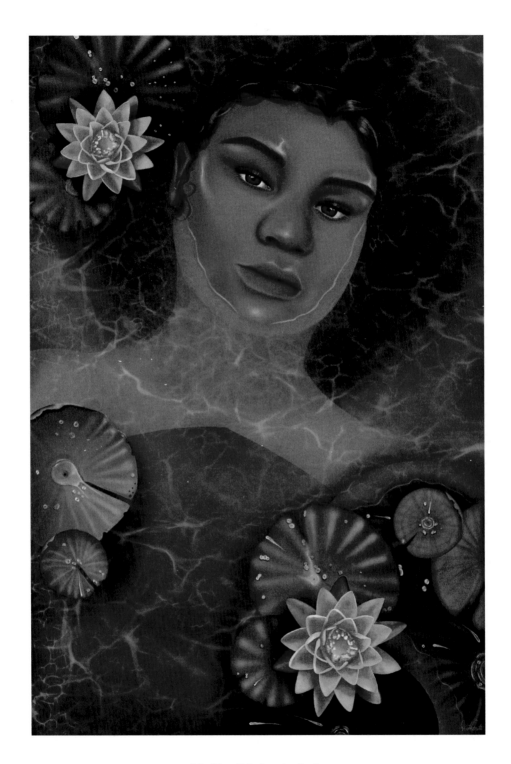

Mud by Cristina Andrade

Graveyard of Misfit Toys

Here is the place where we gather.
We are far from those
Who cast us away.

Here is the place where we heal.
Where not a thing in the world
Dare to harm us.

Here is the place where we belong.
Because there is no other place
We find acceptance.

Here is the place our souls run free
When we shout,
We are heard.

All we've got is each other,
We are one.
There are no
Allies.

We find comfort here.
There is life in us.
There is love.

Once exiled,
Forced to survive,
Now,
We thrive.

We've built ourselves a kingdom.

Rule alongside
Me.

They'd left us to suffer,
Yet we dance,
A family,
We've become.

They dug our graves,
Yet we do not fall.
We are stronger now
That before.

They call this
They graveyard of misfit toys,
But we are not
Broken
Or dying.

You who cursed the name's
Of earth's children,
You who seek refuge after
Your own destruction,
You are not welcome here.

A Drop In The Ocean

I was only

A drop

In the ocean.

I longed

To be

A wave.

I crashed

To shore

To kiss the land.

I gave life

To every

Living thing.

I flow

Effortlessly

As the moon

Whispers to me

Her commands

To the tides.

I caress

Those

Who wish

To dance

With me.

But,

I am mighty.

I am powerful.

I am infinite.

I am confined

To no one

And nothing.

I am limitless

Beyond horizons.

I am bottomless

Beyond imagination.

I am eternal.

I am boundless.

I am constant.

I am enduring.

I am sovereign.

I am dynamic.

I am paramount.

I am complete.

I am free.

I am not

A drop

In the ocean.

I am

The ocean.

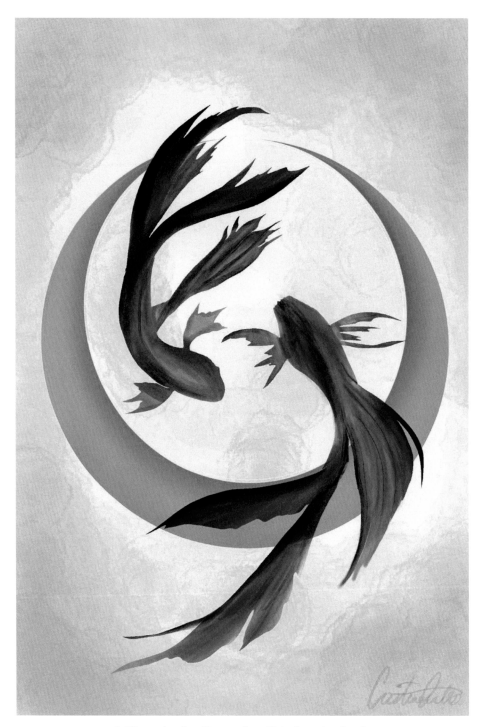

A Drop in the Ocean by Cristina Andrade

Born To Run

Gazelles

Are born running.

They have

No other choice.

Forced

To adapt to being

Prey from the moment

They are born.

Before

The lion can sink

It's teeth into

The gazelle's flesh,

It is too far ahead.

Not

Fleeing for it's

Life, but taking life

Into its own hands

Before it can be taken.

No one

Can tell a gazelle not

To run.

Ketchup Hearts

Mom used to draw

Ketchup hearts

When she made

My lunch.

Mom used to kiss

My forehead

When she told

Me "goodnight."

Mom doesn't make

Sandwiches anymore

And she moved

Far away.

Mom says she's

Got no good

Memories

Here.

She doesn't call

She says I'm not hers

Anymore.

We are on two planets,

In two worlds.

Mom has forgotten

Our ketchup hearts.

Save Them

Save them!

Save them!

Save them!

But

I am a single voice

And I cannot

Save the world.

My voice is but

A whisper in a roar.

My

Voice is weak.

My

Face is cold.

My

Body is worn.

Please

Save them.

Make Me Beautiful

I screamed at the sky

I said "Make me beautiful!"

Suddenly,

I was thin,

I was pale,

I was plastic.

I screamed at the gods

I said, "Make me beautiful!"

Suddenly,

There is stardust in my veins,

Flowers grew from my scalp,

Rivers flowing from my eyes as I wept.

I screamed at the mirror.

I said, "Make me beautiful!"

Suddenly,

I watched ghostly hands rip me apart,

I had measuring tape around my throat,

I straighten my brittle and dead hair.

I whispered to myself.

I said, "Make me beautiful."

And suddenly,

I wasn't thin,

I wasn't pale,

I wasn't plastic.

Suddenly,

There was no stardust,

There were no flowers,

There were no rivers.

Suddenly,

I saw no hands,

I could breathe,

I had new growth.

I whispered to myself.

I said, "Make me beautiful."

And suddenly,

I was.

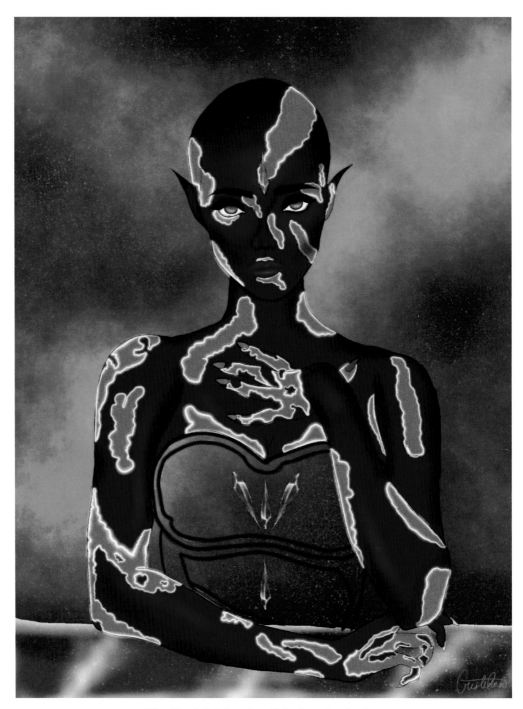

The Deal Maker by Cristina Andrade

<u>I Promise</u>

My body is not
A temple.
It is my kingdom.

My body is not
A war ground.
It is sacred to the earth.

My body is not
A machine.
It is nature's creation.

I dream of being
One with the earth,
One with the elements.

I dream of being
One with the flora,
One with the fauna.

I dream of being
One with my ancestors,
One with the gods.

I dream of being
One with the stars,
One with the ocean.

I will not dare
Touch my skin
With negative intention.

I will not dare
Speak to myself
With negative words.

I will not dare
Surround myself
With negative energy.

I promise
To use my body
For strength
And for growth.

I promise
To use my body
For love
And for trust.

I promise
To use my body
For healing
And for recovery.

I promise
To use my body
For compassion
And for thriving.

Achilles

Below me lies who I was.

Above me, who I will become.

A perpetual dance betwixt them,

My toes along the string of fate

That binds them.

I hold a dagger in one hand,

A parachute in the other.

I feel them.

Lurking, lying in wait.

A sudden stumble.

Shock.

Blood at my heel.

Do I float or fall?

Hero

My grandmother told me
If I wanted to save the world,
I had better save myself.

Stop being a hero.
Hang up the phone.
Cancel plans.
Rest.

Stop pleasing them.
Take my fucking meds.
Put myself first.
Eat.

Stop overworking.
Health comes first.
Don't overdo it.
Hydrate.

Stop neglecting my needs.
Do more than survive.
I deserve better.
Fight.

I can't help them

If I'm not here.

One day at a time.

<u>**"J"**</u>

Jane.
I could have been Jane.

You branded me
With the letter,
With the fate,
With the name.

You said to be
Perfect On Paper.
That's what
Your father wanted.
My lips sewn shut,
Scales nailed to my feet,
Numbers written
On my skin.

Sometimes I wished
I was Jane.
Nameless,
Faceless.

Helpless,

Afraid,

Trapped.

The Letter J tattooed

On my tongue.

Endless night.

In a daze,

Unable to move,

To fight,

To speak.

I lay still,

Watching myself

From above

My own body.

Help her.

Jane told me to get

Justice.

I spoke.

But I was defeated

Before I began.

So, I escaped.

You cannot catch me.

You will not catch me.

Not anymore.

I am free

From the letter J.

I still

Can't say

Your name.

<u>Violet</u>

I saw shades of violet in you

When only red shown.

You shouted, "red!"

When I asked your name.

I didn't hear you.

I asked how you were.

"Violet," you said,

 But you were red.

You had always been red.

Your eyes, ruby.

Your voice, carnelian.

Your hands, maroon.

Red.

Your lips curled up,

Sly and knowing.

"It's your fault you saw violet."

Dancing With Fire

I used to dance with fire.
Flames would frolic
Across my body
With every move.
Sparks would fly
From the tips
Of my fingers.

Volcanoes would weep,
Shaking the earth
To its core,
Filling with the skies
With emotion
For me.

Stars would come to life,
Burning white hot,
Larger than life.
They would rain down
Upon me,
Granting my every wish.
Supernovas
Would applaud me.

I was ablaze.

I would dance

Faster, brighter, hotter.

Until I burned out.

My flames no longer

Frolicking,

My fingertips

No longer spark.

I was cold.

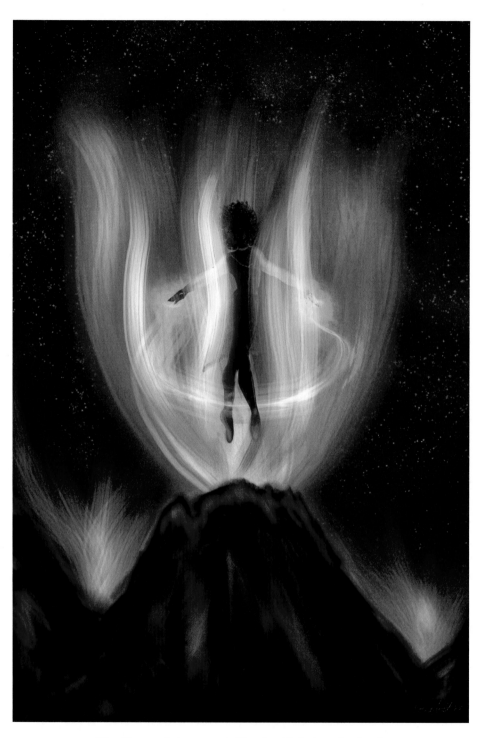

She Danced Amongst Fire by Cristina Andrade

Penguins

The Emperor penguin mates for life.

They choose a mate and

Love them,

Only them,

Until their last,

Dying,

Breath.

A lesson.

We should not

Punish ourselves,

By limiting one another

To the experience of love,

To be loved, only once in this life.

Shed your feathers, take a swim, this love is for you.

Potions

I bought a potion today
To take you away.
Still, you persisted.

As though my torment
Was a national pastime,
You force-fed me poison
And it was televised.

We trade potions
As medicine.
Happiness, growth, education.
We exude love.
This is meditation.

You said we were lucky
We had a place to pray.
Three fires in a week.
Silence where our bodies lay.

When I die, riot for my life.
Ain't enough potions for our strife.

Mosaic

They dare
To tell me my
Skin does not glow
With the sweat and
The blood of my ancestors.

They dare
To tell me my
Hair does not grow
Like the branches of
The tree of life.

They dare
To tell me my
Blood does not flow
Like the oceans that
Kiss the corners of the
Earth from which I am made.

I am a plethora of
Jagged,
Vibrant,
Pieces that fit together

Beautifully.

Breathtakingly.

Spelling out

Shauntia.

My name may cut your tongue,

Taking its vengeance

On those who complain

About the way

It refuses to mold

Itself around your tongue.

It requires effort.

Do it justice,

Or be silent.

I am art

With a dagger.

Armor

My softness
Comes wrapped in armor
Stainless steel and
Amethyst.

No heavier than I
Can handle, for
I do not go
Into battle alone.

I lift my helmet,
Showing my crooked
Teeth, my imperfect skin.
My coiled, umber hair.
My hickory eyes glowing in the sun.

I would show you
The fullness of my body,
The richness of my skin,
The tenderness of my soul,
But you do not deserve it.

Melt

Melt into me.

You have my permission.

You and I,

Forming a marble pillar.

Stronger together,

Twice as beautiful.

Kiss me softly.

Slowly.

With good intentions.

Trace hearts

On my stomach

Show my body

The kindness it deserves.

Melt.

Circles

Looking up from my
Pillow,
Eyes full of fireflies.
I can't keep them open.

My head and my
Gut
Swimming in opposite
Circles.

You said it was fun.
I did a good job.

The days went in
Circles.
I haven't
Exhaled
In
A
Week.

I lose eleven pounds
In that time.

Where are my meds?
I'm talking in
Circles.

I did something
Wrong,
But you won't say what.
We go in
Circles.

I'm dizzy and
Afraid.
You laugh,
It's fun for you.
You like
Circles.

Daffodils

Daffodils,

Precious and gentle.

All wrapped up

For the night,

Protected against

The elements

On this cold,

Endless night.

By morning,

Stretching its petals

Into the sky.

Welcome home.

Architect

She laid brick and mortar

And formed a tower,

Which she called home.

She would look to the sky,

Her only companion,

Making wishes by night,

Singing to the clouds by day.

She's comfortable within her walls.

But she's lonely.

She climbs to the top

To take in the view

Of what she's been keeping at bay.

Magic.

Wonder.

Adventure.

Love.

Loss.

Hope.

She's afraid,

But she climbs down.

She removes one brick.

Then two.

Soon, the world is at her feet.

Her heart is in her throat,

But she's powerful.

She forged a

Sword,

Ready for battle.

Sweat trickles off

The corner of her brow.

Her hands,

Trembling.

She takes a deep breath,

And leaps.

<u>Happy Place</u>

Lay back,

The ground is soft.

The scent of

Lavender

Wafts over you.

Close your eyes.

Stretch out your legs.

Wiggle your toes.

Deep breath in.

1

      2

          3

              4

                    5

                        6

                            7

                                8

                                    9

                                        10

Out.

Stretch your arms,

Flex your hands.

Can you hear the
Waterfall?
Gentle crashes
Upon the rocks.
Deep breath in.
10
          9
            8
               7
                 6
                   5
                     4
                       3
                         2
                           1

Out.
A low,
Warm breeze.
Distant bird calls.
Eyes open.

Black Sappho

I wore my best
Dress,
Lace and Lilac.

I waited beneath
Our favorite tree
To surprise you.

A gentle tap
On the shoulder
And a slow,
Soft, squeeze around
My waist fills me
With butterflies.

I whip around
To hand you a violet
Bouquet I picked for you,
Only to be given one in return.

I cup your face,
Goddess in my hands,
A tear-filled kiss,

Our lips fold up

Into knowing smiles.

I love you.

The world fades

Into shades of

Pink.

All I can see

Is you.

Dear Fat Girl

Beautiful fat girl,
You are deserving
Of love.

Lovely fat girl,
Take up space.
The world is yours.

Powerful fat girl,
Wear it.
You're allowed.

Sexy fat girl,
Treat yourself.

Fat girl,
You matter,
You are worthy
You are a goddess.

They used to make
Statues that look like
You.

You are Venus.

You are

Love.

You

Are

Loved.

Rise

Hand in hand,
Skin to skin
With my sisters.

A sea of gradient
Earth tones.
Brown eyes glowing gold
In the sun.

Mother Earth
Holds us in her hand
And kisses us on
The forehead.
A blessing.

A message to keep going.
That we are loved.
That we can be soft.

Brown girls,
Black girls,
This world is yours.
Rise.

The Color Series

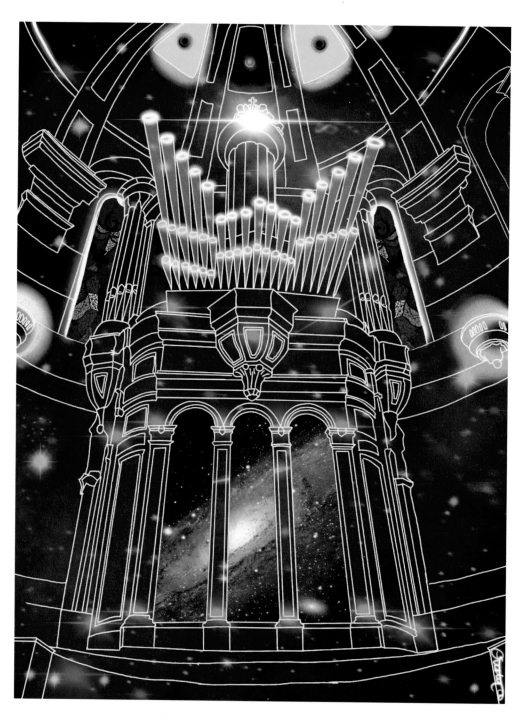

Unnamed by Cristina Andrade

<u>Purple</u>

It is royalty,
It is aura.

It is ancestry,
Nobility,
Luxury.

It is cosmic,
Creative,
Ancient.

It is sensitive,
Mysterious,
Equal.

It is spiritual,
Imagination,
Wealth.

It is art,
Performance,
Intellectuality.

It is imperialism,

Decadence,

Mourning.

It it wisdom,

Diversity,

Balance.

I wonder,

Is it truly

Coincidence

That is is such a

Rarity?

Blue

Cold,
Wet,
Slow,
Denim jeans,
And the sky.

Dark,
Bright,
Electric,
And Robin's egg.

Cleanliness,
Strength,
Authority,
The ocean and
Its mysteries.

Dependability,
Integrity,
Trust,
The sky
Is clear.

Peace,

Depression,

The fiercest

Form of fire.

Serenity,

Infinity,

Loyalty,

Your grandmother's

Eyes.

Protection,

Addiction,

Communication,

The veins running

Through my body.

Devotion,

Nostalgia,

Sincerity,

The color of

My collar.

Depth,

Confidence,

Faith,

Warning: Loss

Of appetite.

Deceitful,

Spiteful,

Unstable,

Always stay under

The radar.

Superstitious,

Predictable,

Unforgiving,

The waves that

Swallow you whole.

Aloof,

Frigid,

Manipulative,

Can I still

Get into Heaven?

Green

Mother Earth,

Tranquility,

Growth,

Nature,

Protect her.

The Green Man,

Fertility,

Rebirth,

Vegetation,

Save him.

The Dynasty,

Heaven,

Luck,

Wealth,

Remember us.

The Great Balancer,

Energy,

Stability,

Recovery,

Heal me.

A Sanctuary,

Harmony,

Renewal,

Relaxation,

Restore them.

The Observer,

Love,

Nature,

Peace,

Just

Listen.

Yellow

Here we come,

With

Optimism,

Happiness,

And Spring!

We come running

With

Education,

Laughter,

And Enlightenment!

Overflowing

With

Hope,

Ideas,

And Courage!

Caution!

Danger!

Alert!

Slow down!

Where have the

Canaries gone?

Suddenly,

We are

Cowardice,

Egoism,

And toxic!

Suddenly,

We are

Impulsive,

Venomous,

And impatient!

There once were many

Of us,

Golden,

Citrin,

And cream.

There once were many

Of us,

Lonely,

Fickle,

And curious.

There once were many
Of us,
Melancholy,
Sensitive,
And Cynic.

There once were many
Of us,
But there was
Not enough of
The paint
For the rest of us.

Orange

I
Am what
The sun sets in.

I
Am what
Lives in fire.

I
Am what
Keeps you warm.

I
Am your
Vitamin C.

I
Am your
Warnings.

I
Am your
Health.

I

Give

Life.

I

Give

Purpose.

I

Give

Vitality.

I

Am

Vibrance

I

Am

Hazard.

I

Am

Sacred.

I
Am
Humanity.

Red

It is passion,

It is strength,

It is fury.

It is anger,

It is lust,

It is adventure.

It is seduction,

It is danger,

It is history.

It is power,

It is blood,

It is heroism.

It is hatred,

It is war,

It is magic.

It is prosperity,

It is the equilibrium,

It is fire.

It is pain,
It is pleasure,
It is pure energy.
It is determination,
It is visibility,
It is intensity.

It is ambition,
It is intelligence.
It is maturity.

It is the heart,
It is beauty,
It is love.

You look so good
In red.

Guest Poems

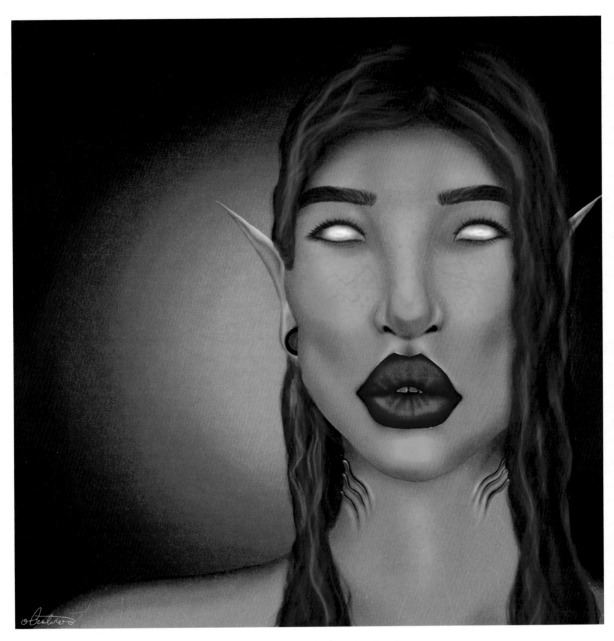

Beckoning by Cristina Andrade

Struggle

By @apathetic.alicorn on instagram

Pain, disability, isolation.

Clarity, enlightenment, and faith.

Being disabled is a double bladed sword,

Allowing me to greatful, and also angry.

Thanks to the system that fucks us over,

Thankful for the people who support me

Throughout everything.

Chronic pain is a curse and

A blessing,

Showing me life's colors,

The many shades of grey.

Chronic pain shows me

Who truly cares and who doesn't.

And for that, I'm eternally grateful.

Beckoning

By Cristina Andrade

I've never understood the premise of color

On some days, I wake up and my skin is blue and my eyes are red

Beckoning

On these days there are fine lines etched into my skin that tell the story of a race of beings I have never met

On other days my skin shines like sand dunes in summer,

There exist scars and scratches of the battles where I have been victorious

On days where my skin is ash and my eyes are green there lies sigils
etched into my flesh of spells and curses that have been cast upon me

And like colors I don't understand I rub distance into my skin to throw their words back

And suddenly I'm brand new

a blank slate of a million colors and sounds that dance into their
tones around me

Beckoning

the colors etch into me
Teach me to dance, to sing, to hear
and their color is a melody I'll never need to tune

routine.

By Rhiannon Moline (@rhiammon on instagram)

name.

date of birth.

address.

how are you feeling today?

on a scale of one to ten?

does that hurt?

oh no.

ordering more tests.

no need to worry.

name.

date of birth.

address.

how are you feeling today?

on a scale of one to ten?

can you go like this?

down to floor four.

don't worry.

everything is fine.

name.

date of birth.

address.

how are you feeling today?

on a scale of one to ten?

are the meds working?

up the dose.

side effects may include.

you'll be okay.

name.

date of birth.

address.

how are you feeling today?

on a scale of one to ten?

again?

just one more.

then you're done.

wonderful job.

name.

date of birth.

address.

stop.

please.

Untitled

Kelsey B (@kelthulu on instagram)

This feeling eats at my bones.

I grind against myself

And will my body to move against the rust that builds on My face.

My legs.

My arms.

I smile at them gently,

But despite what everyone says

No amount of warm disposition has ever melted the ice that has

left me

Frozen where I stand.

he?

By @aa_poetry_ on instagram

have i ever met someone who deserves for me to drown for him? toss myself into stinging waves and hold my breath as i sink to the bottom?

then swim upward, force myself through the vigorous currents, find myself at the surface and tear every inch of my skin off as i scramble up an ash grey cliff to meet with him on dry land?

has someone crossed my path who i'd put to death my dreams for, watch the scrolls i scrawl my art upon burn to dust in a glaring haze before my tearful eyes?

would i have ever allowed my knees to tremble and shiver until they gave way and brought me to the feet of any man who has crossed my path? has anyone been worthy of the passion i could give him?

was the boy with the face made of fool's gold worth the kingly title of "first crush?" was there anything beyond his unrelieved mediocrity which proved such divinity? by what quality did he have the arrogance to claim such a position? in what state of tragic intoxication was i to knight him so?

Did the boy who crawled into my fantasies with his eyes closed so much as speak a word to me to prove that he is the mesmerising tapestry i once saw elegantly sewn into his skin? was there at all any sweet, sweet melody i heard flow through his rugged voice that i danced to at midnight and swore by my life i could hear? by what miseducation did i find it necessary to take it upon myself to hang him in the louvre?

and the one in whom i found some miraculous delight, could i have ever found painted underneath a halo? was he, as i had hastily concluded, the answer to my desperate cries? did the conversations made of self deprecating banter, comically harsh slander and outright vomiting our dreams into the sky promise a chance to live among the stars? was he worth every exception, the energy it took to plaster his face onto the body that i might one day have the mind to take a bullet for and pretend that it isn't obviously photoshop?

was he? was he? was he?

and if, by the chance that my newspaper horoscope prediction allows, i find myself one day gazing into the gleaming eyes of someone i might be able to write a love poem about one day, will he be worth my misery? my crawling naked through the rain whilst crying, my arms aching underneath the weight of his sorrows, my

bones cracking and collapsing upon one another as i make
sacrifice after sacrifice to exist only for him? will he?

Through The Mist

By Joshua Ortiz

Through the mist, I can see your face
The prettiest eyes staring back at me
Your words, they linger and haunt
Hover in the air like a melody

You don't have to do much
Your very presence is more than enough
To mark a change in the atmosphere
To cast away every single fear

Through the fog, I can see your smile
Precious laughter lighting up the room
Your kiss, it leaves me breathless
But you pull away, end it all too soon

I don't know what else I could say
You've changed my life in inconceivable ways
My darkest days have all turned crystal clear
Everything you give, I'm holding so dear
I'm hoping you'll stay
That you're warmed by the fire
And these words, I'm hoping they'll reach you
That your love they'll inspire.

The Artist

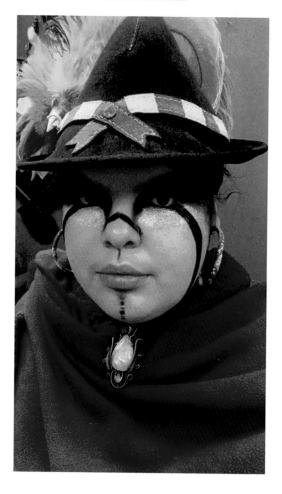

Cristina Andrade is an accomplished artist, musician, activist, and collegiate student who is currently studying Astrophysics. Her life is colored by her childhood in Miami, the many road trips and adventures throughout her life, and her recent move to the midwest. If you'd like to see more of her art, please visit @artofthebanddragonz on instagram.

The Author

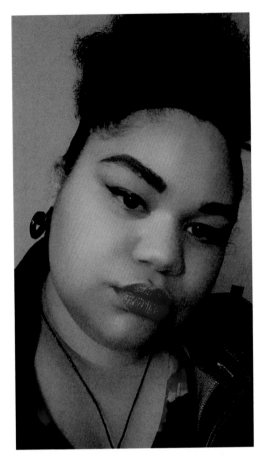

Shauntia Cunningham is a mixed-black twenty-two year old who has used her difficult life experiences to inspire her writing. She grew up in a small village in Ohio and is currently focusing on a degree in forensic psychology. As an activist, she uses her experience to help raise awareness for others. She is currently active on instagram as @chronic.lotus and twitter as @amethystisbii.

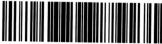

40326589R00050

Made in the USA
Lexington, KY
28 May 2019